Anti-atherosclerotic measures

Constantin Panow

COPYRIGHT 2020

All rights reserved.

"The art of healing comes from nature, not from the physician. Therefore, the physician must start from Nature, with an open mind."
Paracelsus (1494-1541)

DISCLAIMER

This small text cannot replace a visit at the doctor's office. Consult your physician, nutritionist, and personal trainer if you have any medical problem!

CONTENT

Copyright 2020
Disclaimer
Introduction
Political incentive
Imaging
Therapy
Arterial pressure
Others
Fallacies
Diabetes mellitus
Morbid obesity
Fats
Starch Carbohydrates
Fiber Carbohydrates
Meat
Latitude
Paradox
Sports
Different activities
"Step Track"
Resveratrol
Allicin
Drinking water
Essential Fatty Acids

Proposal
Seafood
Diseases
Atherosclerosis
Antioxidants
Nutrition
Arterial Hypertension
Website

INTRODUCTION

Atherosclerosis is main death promoter all over the World.

First cause is arterial hypertension, which is treated most efficiently with drug prescription by your doctor.

Another important factor is tobacco.

POLITICAL INCENTIVE

Those two have been combatted very efficiently in recent years by authority and that is why we witness much less this disease for two decades.

Eviction of smoking from public closed spaces, nicotine chewing gums and electronic cigarettes have been all important factors in this struggle.

Publicity makes people more aware of this problem, and once they have grasped the right decision, it is easy to resort to further measures.

Besides, apart from heart infarction, cerebral stroke and peripheral arterial obliteration, tobacco is a strong cancer promoter.

IMAGING

As a radiologist, I have been amazed twenty years ago how important arterial intima plaque calcifications were.

Those are simple calcium depositions on inner arterial wall.

THERAPY

To solve this issue, nothing but chemistry can help.

As with rocks, especially limestone, dissolved in rain, acid introduced in the body can do.

Lemon juice, which is citric acid, dissolves prostate stones.

Vinegar, which is acetic acid, is known since centuries for its positive properties on human health.

Populations consuming a lot of it live longer than surrounding ones.

Here we should discuss the way of introducing acid in one's body.

Lemon dissolves also teeth enamel, if brought in direct touch with it.

Result is tooth caries!

Thus, you should dilute the juice and drink it through a straw.

As, to vinegar, I like to dilute it in water 1/3 to 2/3 about, and when I am used to it, even half-half.

Populations consuming a lot vinegar enjoy a longer life expectancy.

ARTERIAL PRESSURE

I season it with salt. As I suffer from arterial hypotension, I love salt and eat quantities of it.

Of course, if you suffer from arterial hypertension, this makes a difference.

Consult your physician beforehand and measure your arterial tension regularly!

OTHERS

In the same way pickles and other vegetables prepared in vinegar are extremely healthy products. If you find them too sour, it is easy to wash them in water before consumption.

Winter salad: red peppers 1 kg, green peppers 1 kg, bell peppers 1 kg, carrots 1 kg, green tomatoes 1 kg, cauliflower 1 kg, cabbage 1 kg, celery 1 kg, heads, stalks, and leaves. Souse, brine: water 2 l, vinegar 1 l, vegetal oil 50 ml, salt 300 g, honey 500 g, bay leaves, black pepper. You boil the brine, and once boiling, you pour it over the vegetables.

The next day you take away the brine and you bring it to boiling again. You pour it again over the vegetables, and you leave it resting in a cool place overnight. The next day it should be ready for consuming. If not, you can wait two or three days longer.

Spring salad: Boiled spring potatoes with pealing, spring onions, pickles, olives, dill, salt, water, mayonnaise, vegetal oil, and lemon or vinegar.

Many more recipes contain lemon and vinegar.

Romans would give this last one to Gladiators, diluted in salty water.

It is an excellent thirst quencher in hot summer

days.

Apart from that well-known is use of both acids in salad seasonings.

Be it green salad, ripe tomatoes, cucumbers, or peppers.

These last ones I prefer to grill first, wrap them in paper, and peal them when they have cooled down.

I season them with vinegar or lemon juice, salt, and colza oil.

By the way, do not forget to add some water in every salad sauce!

Avocados, in the same way, we prepare with lemon, salt and mayonnaise.

Well known in the Middle East is the beverage Ajran.

I prepare it with yoghurt, lemon juice and salt, diluted in a bit of water. This way you do not need to drink through a straw.

Green beans I like to boil first, then take them out of the water and put them in the frying pan with oil until they are well cooked, and at last add some lemon with salt.

In a plate of cooked old beans, or lentils, I like to add vinegar and colza oil.

Gazpacho is a cold summer soup, prepared in a blender: onion, ripe tomatoes, cucumber, dill, lemon or vinegar, salt, and pepper, all mixed together.

Tarama I prepare also in a blender: spring onions, dill, salty cod roe, water, a lot of vegetal oil, and lemon or vinegar.

Fish once cooked we season with a lot of lemon.

This is particularly useful for smoked salmon.

There is a dish in South America, which is called Seviche-raw fish left in lemon juice overnight. This is of course an attempt to kill the parasites.

Cirros salad: This is dried spring mackerel, (as autumn one is too greasy for this purpose). You grill shortly the fish to sterilize it. Then you hammer it into small pieces. It should be washed in water to take away the salt excess. You season it in water and vegetal oil, vinegar, or lemon, and dill, and you can eat it after a few hours.

FALLACIES

During the fifties of last century, there emerged an opinion in the States that fat should be responsible for atherosclerosis.

It appeared recently that this is wrong and from dangerous nutritional factors the main one is sugar.

DIABETES MELLITUS

This disease is very deleterious for blood vessels.

MORBID OBESITY

This one results from faulty nutrition, with an excess of meat, sugars, and starches.

Result is most frequently diabetes type 2.

FATS

On the other hand, olive oil, butter, and animal fat are even beneficial for atherosclerosis, protecting vessel walls against it.

If not consumed in excess those ones permit to slim down.

STARCH CARBOHYDRATES

Bread, pasta, potatoes, rice, and other cereals, having a high glycemic index, should not be consumed in excessive amounts.

Remains unclear the role of lectins, gluten, and alimentary intolerances and allergies.

To my opinion they also play a role in atherosclerosis.

FIBER CARBOHYDRATES

Eating more vegetables protects your arteries.

Fruit has also a positive effect. Prefer small one, like blackberries, blueberries, raspberries, and strawberries, as they are rich in polyphenols!

MEAT

Avoid too much meat in your diet. Our ancestors would eat it twice per year only, pork at Christmas and lamb at Easter.

Prefer rather poultry and even better fish, as those species are much farther away from our own constitution!

LATITUDE

Arterial hypertension depends largely on sun exposition.

Hence this illness is rare around the Equator, with a prevalence increasing toward the poles.

Stress hormones also play an important role in it. Thus, if you lack sunshine, take some vitamin D instead!

PARADOX

Eskimos, called also Innuits, as they eat meat and fish raw, would suffer little during first half of last century from vascular diseases.

This was a big dilemma for 50 years, until we understood the role of vitamin D and essential fats as protectors.

SPORTS

Regular exercise is also important for prevention of atherosclerotic disease. Most important is walking. Medical books advertise one whole hour each day.

DIFFERENT ACTIVITIES

Endurance training, which is exercising the aerobic system seems to extenuate the body, and we observe sometimes tremendous vascular disease with it.

Opposed to this one is strength training, which exercises the anaerobic system. We advertise this one instead.

Another advantage also of this last one, is that with aerobics attained proficiency fades away quickly. In one or two weeks you must start all over again.

Anaerobic acquisitions last much longer, even up to several years.

Weightlifting gives fast results on the short term but ends up with articulation problems with time.

That is why I prefer calisthenics. Limiting training to bodyweight has the least negative effect on joints.

I enjoy several sets of pushups per day.

Famous trainers propose quarter of an hour Cardio six days of the week.

If you observe hygiene rules of this one, as for instance heart rate, such a measure seems extremely wise.

"Step Track"

Squats are dangerous for your knees.

I replace them with a variation which I call the "Step Track".

You lean with the back against a wall, legs bent at 90°, and you change weight from one leg to the other.

This one should be executed on tip toes, to exercise your calf's muscles as well. If you suffer from meniscus tear, you should do it only on heels.

RESVERATROL

France is a country well known for its cuisine.

Most people know high quality French wines and cheese, best valued in the whole world.

Few know that French people are between the healthiest in the World, with the longest life expectancy in Europe.

Many relate this fact to joyous character of French people, with high alcohol consumption.

Especially Resveratrol in red wine is well known for its vascular protective properties.

A patient in my consultation proposed to my questioning eyes that he was practicing the triathlon:

Red and white wine and rosé!

ALLICIN

Garlic is another product, which protects vascular integrity. Beware, cooking neutralizes it.

Bringing it above 70°C renders it inefficient.

This is not the only positive effect of this product. It has anti-infective properties, especially against mold and fungus.

DRINKING WATER

Hardness of water is inversely proportional to atherosclerosis. That is people who are drinking for years water which has been rendered sweeter (softer) by ion-exchange suffer from atherosclerotic disease. High content of calcium carbonate ($CaCO_3$) in drinking water protects against atherosclerosis.

ESSENTIAL FATTY ACIDS

Many tissues in human body are composed of a lot of membranes. As a matter of fact, all cells are limited by one.

Main constituent are lipids.

Nutrition in modern society is largely deficient in essential fatty acids. Since half a century physician recommend Olive Oil. This one contains Omega 9, but no 3 and 6.

PROPOSAL

For Omega 3 you need Linen Oil, possibly cold-pressed, and for Omega 6 Safflower Oil. Last one is a small cactus and there is no way to extract fat from it without heating.

Sunflower and Colza oil contain both acids, but to variable proportions.

Supplementation of those products can prevent a lot of diseases.

As all liquids in the body in inappropriate location tend to be resorbed, we can hope that such a treatment could help also reversing illnesses.

As for instance, in dissection of vertebral artery, which is a very delicate issue, we do not apply for the moment other therapy than Aspirin, with full success in many cases.

I recommend Linen and Safflower oil, three teaspoons each daily.

In case of non -availability or intolerance one can resort to colza, or sunflower oils, possibly cold-pressed.

Add it to salad and vegetables to ease absorption!

SEAFOOD

Fish contains Omega 3, but as soon you cook it, it is gone.

Cooling the stuff near 0°C or below has probably the same effect as heating it.

Hence, vegetal oils should be kept at about 10-15°C, away from daylight, and for not longer than 10 months, to avoid deterioration.

In this last case the stuff becomes neither healthy nor tasty.

During the cold season you can consume seafood raw, but from warmer waters it is infested with parasites, which on the long-term cause liver cancer.

DISEASES

Probably many ailments have as a common origin a deficit in essential fatty acids.

(Fissures in tendons, arterial aneurysms, dissections, and arterio-venous malformations, adenomyosis and endometriosis, cataract, retinal detachment, vertebral discus herniation, neuropathy, Barlow's disease, cardiac Arrhythmias, and many more.)

Main target are structures composed of very long cells, which means a huge load of membranes. Fundamental constituents of those ones are lipids.

Their thus central ingredients prevent cells from decay and sloughing.

Adding Vitamin A accelerates restauration of involved organs.

I recommend whole oranges, one per day, to be pealed, but eaten with the white part, as this helps digestion.

French people say that this fruit is Gold at breakfast, Silver at lunch and Lead at supper.

ATHEROSCLEROSIS

As mentioned previously, this disease is most common in aging population. Prevalence is huge, which renders it most frequent killer on Earth.

Heart infarction, stroke, peripheral arterial occlusions are the result.

Its etiology is manyfold, but main one is deficit in essential fatty acids. Endothelial cells are long ones with a lot of membrane.

This one needs several components for its constitution.

In deficit of essential fatty acids attempt at its construction ends up with excess of cholesterol, another constituent, which forms an inordinate plaque.

Thus, limiting endothelium decays leaving a gap, open to blood flow.

A scar is then striving to bridge it. Undue Collagen 1 and 3 builds on it.

As it remains naked, osteoblasts infiltrate this newly apposed tissue, and calcification starts.

This happens in analogy to bone, where no

endothelium is needed.

As this newly formed matrix is subjected to compression forces from pulsating vessel wall, even unwarranted ossification takes place.

All this process needs energy, which is supplied by body stores.

Glucose gives up Pyruvate, a molecule with two Oxygen atoms, each with one free «minus» valence. Hence, Oxidation occurs easily with this source.

This is much less pronounced with lipid metabolism, where energy product is a Ketonic body, a molecule with two saturated Oxygen atoms, without free valences.

ANTIOXIDANTS

This is where Antioxidants intervene. Those are present in fruit and vegetables. Small fruit contains the most: Cranberry, Raspberry, Blueberry, Strawberry, BlackBerry, Boysen Berry, Lingon Berry, Elder Berry.

Those ones encompass favorable acids also, which dissolve Calcium Carbonate and Phosphate crystals.

Season fruit and vegetables are less expensive, and worthwhile than the one coming from far away.

This last is uneconomical and means a huge kerosene load and CO_2 release on the Globe.

In last decade brands abound, which propose antioxidants in pills.

Few useful addresses are for instance Bilberry Extract (https://pureclinica.com), Curcumasan and Schwarzer Knoblauch (www.alpinamed.ch).

NUTRITION

As you can notice from previous expose, food which promotes atherosclerosis is on the side of sugars and starches, rather than fats.

Also, eating big quantity protein is not healthy, as excess converts immediately into glucose.

Modern nutrition proposes for lipids consuming half saturated and the other fifty percent unsaturated ones.

As a considerable number Omega acids have been described, it is useful swapping vegetal oils.

Also, inclusion of nuts in one's diet is exceedingly healthy. Those ones contain apart from essential fatty acids microelements present in small measure in other food.

Walnuts, pecans, cashews, hazelnuts, peanuts, macadamia nuts, pine nuts, Brazil nuts, pistachios, butternuts, and others.

In some cases, kernels of apricots are sweet, and taste like almonds. Discard the bitter ones, as they enclose cyanide, most powerful poison in nature.

Pumpkin seeds and other can be included in one's diet.

One handful of nuts is the usually prescribed daily portion.

Some are difficult to obtain at an acceptable price. An address I use for pine tree nuts, "Bio Pinienkernmus" is (https://www.koro-shop.ch).

ARTERIAL HYPERTENSION

This is the associated killer. It is less common in areas with high sun exposure. Obviously, Vitamin D load plays a central role.

Its appearance is tightly linked with atherosclerosis.

Blood pressure receptors in arterial walls, for instance the carotid sinus, do not transmit absolute measures for feed-back to the kidneys.

They only register the difference between systolic and diastolic levels.

Hence, if elasticity of vessel façade is reduced, as in atherosclerosis, kidneys retain more liquid and salt.

I hope you enjoyed this short text.

WEBSITE

You can join me at the:
www.thenopillshealthprospect.com
If you have questions or comments, do not hesitate, write in my blog!

www.ingramcontent.com/pod-product-compliance
Lightning Source LLC
Chambersburg PA
CBHW072238230526
45466CB00025B/2104